Pre-Scissor Skills

Skill Starters for Motor Development

Third Editio

by Marsha Dunn Klein, M.Ed., O.T.R.

Illustrations drawn under contract by
Corwyn Zimbleman

Therapy Skill Builders™ 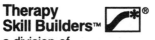®
a division of
The Psychological Corporation

555 Academic Court
San Antonio, Texas 78204-2498
1-800-228-0752

Duplicating

You may prefer to copy the designated reproducible materials by using stencils or spirit masters. Make a single photocopy of the desired page. Use that photocopy to make a stencil or spirit master on a thermal copier.

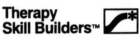
10 9 8 7 6 5 4
Printed in the United States of America

About the Author

After receiving the B.S. degree in Occupational Therapy from Sargent College of Allied Health Professions at Boston University and a Master's in Education from the University of Arizona, **Marsha Dunn Klein** worked with developmentally disabled and physically handicapped persons at the Arizona Training Program for five years. In 1980 she received a Neurodevelopmental Treatment Certificate in pediatrics. Currently she is in private practice as a pediatric therapist in Tucson, Arizona.

Other materials by Marsha Dunn Klein, M.Ed., O.T.R.:
Pre-Dressing Skills
Pre-Sign Language Motor Skills
Pre-Writing Skills
Developmental Position Stickers
Feeding Position Stickers
Feeding Techniques for Children Who Have Cleft Lip and Palate

With Suzanne Evans Morris, Ph.D.:
Pre-Feeding Skills: A Comprehensive Resource for Feeding Development

With Avtar Dunaway, O.T.R.:
Bathing Techniques for Children Who Have Cerebral Palsy
Writing Techniques and Adaptations for Home and Classroom

With Nancy J. Harris, O.T.R.:
Baby Position Stickers
Neonatal Position Stickers

Contents

Introduction

Cutting with scissors can and should be fun! Teachers, parents, and therapists should strive to provide positive learning experiences when teaching this skill to preschool children and developmentally delayed students.

We all learn new tasks in stages, or developmental steps. First we learn the easy parts of a task, and then we build on those skills to learn the more complex parts of the activity. If we do not learn the basics, later we will be frustrated when we are expected to perform the complex steps. When we are frustrated, we quickly lose interest in learning.

In this workbook, the developmental stages of scissor usage are explained. By properly assessing the skill level of each student before initiating a task, we can begin teaching at the student's current level of performance.

We also must provide any adaptations that are necessary for the student to succeed at the new task. Some scissor adaptations are included here.

The workbook is designed to be a tool for independent study. Objectives are specified, and a post-test enables you to assess your information gain. Periodic probes help you to reinforce the information you have just read.

Enjoy the workbook! I hope the variety of activities presented here will help you teach creative scissor skills in your classroom.

Objectives

By the end of this workbook, the reader will be able to:

1. List ten prerequisites for cutting.

2. List the developmental stages of cutting.

3. Name three types of paper that can be used in scissor practice, ranking them in the order of difficulty.

4. Describe three pre-scissor experience games.

5. List four factors to be considered when selecting scissors for an individual student.

6. Describe four (or more) types of scissors.

7. List three adaptations that can help a student who tears paper or bends it in the scissors.

8. Describe four (or more) adaptations that can be used to increase scissor control.

9. Name six (or more) classroom scissor activities that can enhance scissor coordination.

1 Prerequisite Skills for Success in Scissor Usage

Before we examine the specific prerequisite skills necessary to ensure success in the task of cutting with scissors, we must spend some time looking at how children develop and how they normally acquire new motor skills.

Five Principles of Motor Skill Development

Principle 1 Children develop motor skills in a *cephalo-caudal* direction. In other words, they develop control of movements in a head-to-toe direction. They learn head control and shoulder control before walking or fine motor skills are achieved.

Principle 2 Control of movements is gained in a *proximal-to-distal* direction. This means that children learn to control the joints closest to the body (proximal) before being able to control the joints farthest away from the body (distal). They learn to reach and control shoulder movement before achieving elbow, wrist, and finger control.

Principle 3 *Stability* must be achieved before mobility or controlled distal movements are possible. Infants gain control of their shoulders through the process of lying on the tummy and moving their weight from side to side and forward and backward. Control is further refined as the infant crawls and creeps on all fours. We know that stability is being developed because we can see the infant reaching in more and more controlled ways with arms held farther away from the midline. As the shoulders gain stability, the weight-bearing and weight-shifting activities in the elbows and wrists help to refine that more distal control. Now the child can sit and turn the forearms to play with toys in a palm-up or supinated position. As forearm skill is achieved, the child continues to practice grasping a variety of objects with different sizes and shapes from a variety of positions. Children will hold objects in one side of their hands (mobile side) while they creep on the floor with weight on the other side of their hands (stable side).

Principle 4 First movements are "whole body" movements. Later, the child learns to *disassociate* or separate the movements of one particular part of the body. Young infants first "reach" with both arms, legs, eyes, and even the mouth! Gradually they learn to separate their movements so one arm, the legs, and the mouth can rest quietly as the other arm effectively reaches. In grasping, first the whole hand is used. All fingers do the same thing at the same time. Gradually, children learn to move the thumb separately and in opposition to the fingers and to use fingers separately for the refined demands of precise grasping.

Principle 5   Children must pay attention to *survival* issues first. If they are unbalanced and feel as if they may fall off the chair, they will put their attention to their seating rather than to the fine motor task being taught. If they are hungry, sick, or uncomfortable, these sensations will demand their attention.

Ten Prerequisites for Learning to Use Scissors

With an understanding of these five principles, we are ready to look at some specific prerequisites to successful scissors usage. Some of these skills may be missing in children who have physical or sensorimotor difficulties. For these children, instruction and equipment can be adapted in some of the ways presented later in this book.

Prerequisite 1   **Balance**

The child must be able to sit in an upright posture, with feet placed firmly on the floor or on a stool or footrest. The child must be comfortable and have no fear of tipping over. Attention then will be freed to focus on the task of learning to use scissors.

Prerequisite 2   Shoulder Stability

The ability to stabilize and control the movement of the shoulders is important for direct reaching and to provide support for the forearm, wrist, and finger actions required in cutting. The child must be able to control both shoulders so that the arms can perform separate actions without losing precision.

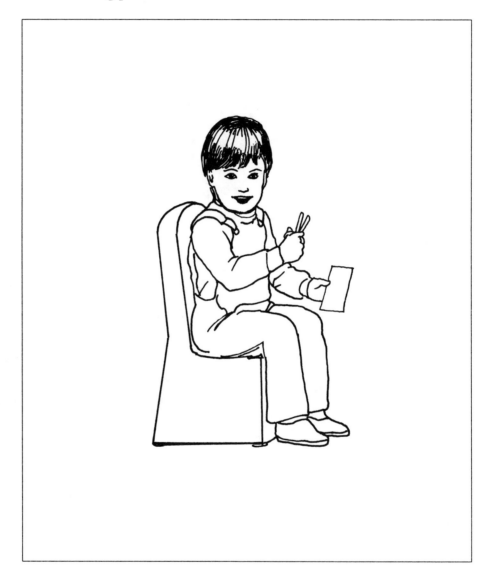

Prerequisite 3 Forearm Control

The child must be able to comfortably move the forearms from a palm-down (pronated) position to a thumb-up (neutral) position to a palm-up (supinated) position. Not only must the child have the range of motion necessary to achieve these movements, but the movements must be done smoothly and with control.

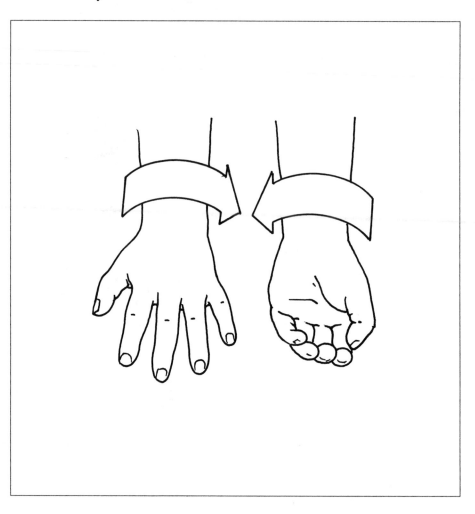

Prerequisite 4 Wrist Stability

The child must be able to hold the wrists in a controlled position and to gradually move them into and out of that stable position. When using two hands for cutting, the wrists each move separately in a graded or controlled way. One hand, holding the paper, moves in one direction while the other hand, holding the scissors, moves in a different manner.

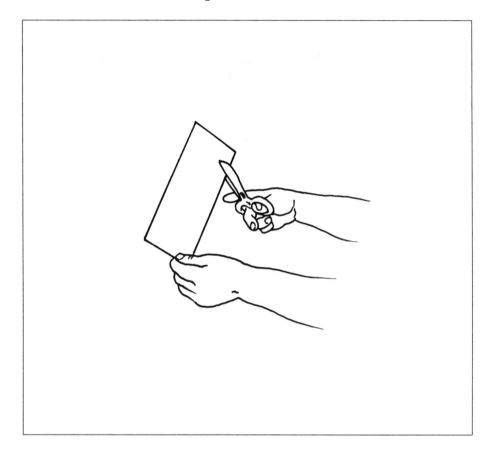

Prerequisite 5   Grasp

The ability to close the hand in the cutting motion is required. One hand must hold the paper, using a grasp on the radial (thumb) side of the hand. The other hand must be able to use the thumb, index finger, and middle finger to control the scissors while the other side of the hand is stabilized.

Prerequisite 6   Finger Isolation

The ability to isolate the action of the thumb, middle finger, and the index finger allows the child to control the opening and closing of the scissor blades. To isolate each finger into a separate action requires considerable control.

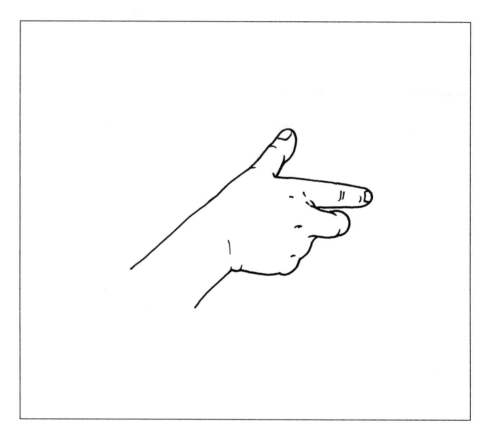

Prerequisite 7   Release

The ability to release an object from the hand is important when grasping the scissors and the paper. It also is part of the action in cutting. First the child "grasps" to close the hand, and then "releases" to open the hand. This results in the up-and-down cutting motion of the scissors.

Prerequisite 8   Lead-Assist Two-Hand Usage

This is the ability to use both hands together, with one hand stabilizing while the other hand leads in the action. It usually requires hand preference to be at least emerging. Actually, the stabilizing (paper-holding) hand must be slightly active as the lead hand moves to perform the cutting actions around corners and angles. This further complicates the task of cutting.

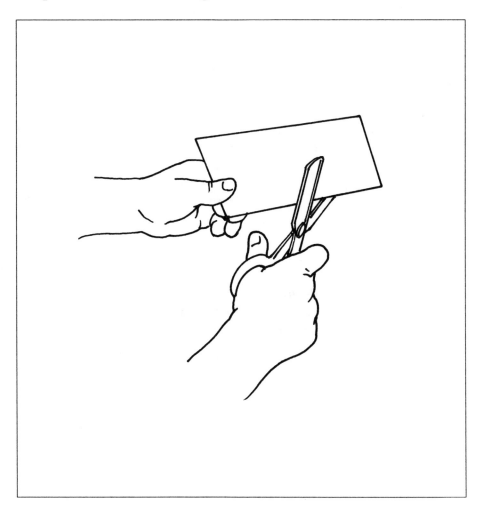

Prerequisite 9 Coordination of Arm, Hand, and Eye Movements

The ability to coordinate the eyes with the finely graded actions of the shoulders, elbows, forearms, wrists, and fingers is required before the child can learn to cut.

Prerequisite 10 Developmental Readiness

Children go through various stages when they are learning to play and interact with their environment. One of the earliest stages can be called the sensory explorative stage, in which the body itself is the child's toy. In this stage, children learn how to move their body parts, to isolate reach and grasp, and to coordinate those skills with vision. Mouthing, reaching, grasping, dropping, shaking, banging, and throwing dominate this stage.

Gradually, interest turns to learning how toys work. Cause-and effect toys then become the most interesting. Children develop specific pushing, pulling, poking, turning, and rolling skills. They explore new toys by dumping them out and taking them apart.

Finally, children enter the constructive stage of play. The take-apart skills of the previous transitional stage make way for filling, building, stacking, and putting together. Instead of seeing objects as a "whole," children begin to notice and interact with the parts. They begin to understand shapes, sizes, colors, and concepts that show relationships of parts. Attention span increases, and children now are ready to scribble, draw, do puzzles, string beads, and be introduced to scissors.

PROBE

Name five principles of normal development that influence the refinement of movements.

List ten prerequisites for scissor usage.

10

2 Developmental Stages of Scissor Usage

As in most tasks of childhood, the ability to master scissor skills proceeds in a sequential pattern of development. Preschool children who are learning to use scissors will quickly pass from unrefined movements to precise skills. Developmentally or physically delayed children, adolescents, or adults may spend more time learning each developmental step, and it may be necessary for teachers or parents to modify either the method or the equipment used.

Learning Initial Skills

Stage 1   **The student shows an interest in scissors.**

The student must show an interest in scissors by bringing scissors to paper or imitating cutting actions with scissors. If the prerequisite motor and developmental play skills are present, the student is ready to learn basic scissor skills.

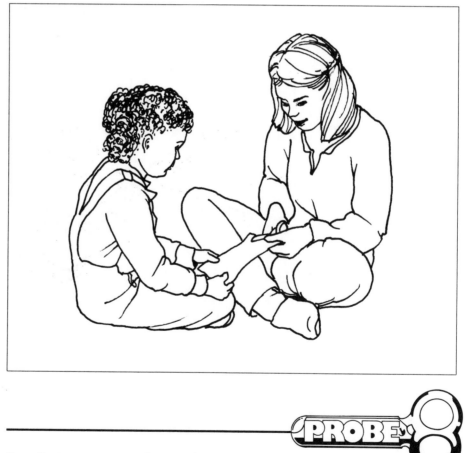

PROBE

In what ways may the student indicate the desire to learn to use scissors?

Stage 2   The student holds and manipulates scissors appropriately.

Next, the student will learn to hold the scissors appropriately. Holding the scissors involves isolating the middle finger and thumb for insertion into the scissor loops, stabilizing the lower loop with the index finger, and resting the scissor loops near the bent middle joints of the fingers.

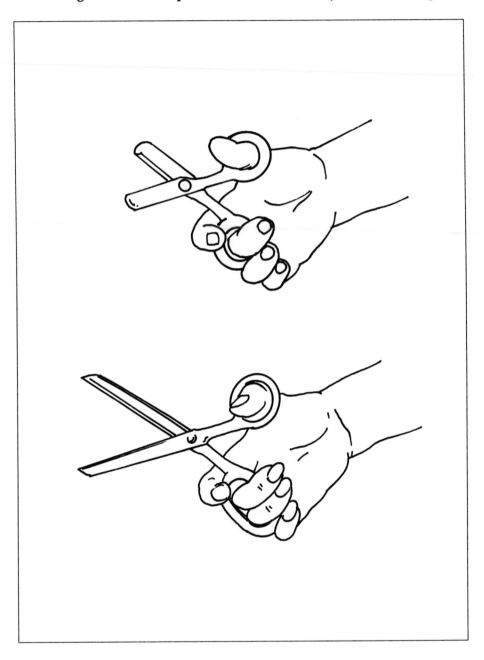

Students sometimes hold the scissors incorrectly in these ways:

No fingers in loops

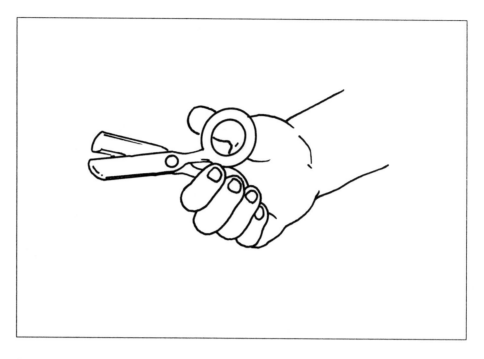

Two-hand approach

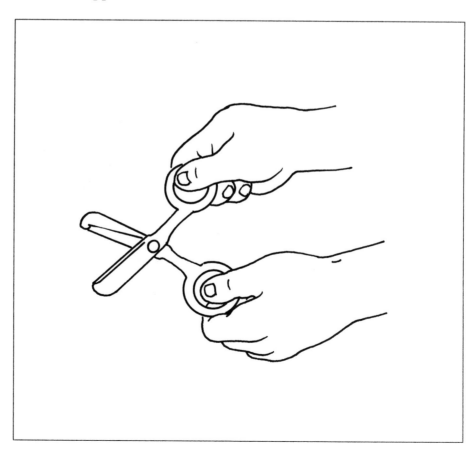

Index and middle fingers in loops

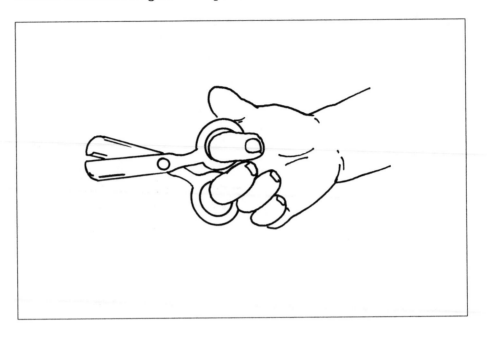

Scissor loops too close to knuckles

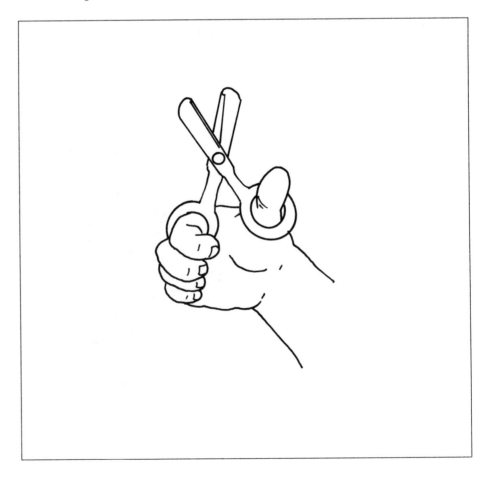

Stage 3 The student opens and closes scissors in a controlled fashion.

After learning to hold the scissors appropriately, the student practices opening and closing the scissors. At this point, there is no need to introduce paper. If you do use paper, don't push the student to cut on lines or in any one direction. The student probably is not yet able to coordinate the motions into a direct cut.

The pre-scissor games on pages 33-36 provide opportunities to practice opening and closing motions.

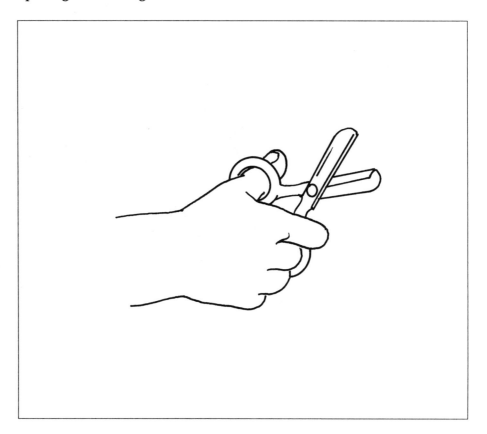

Stage 4 The student cuts short random snips.

Once the student has shown an interest in cutting, has learned to hold the scissors appropriately, and can open and close the scissors in a controlled fashion, it is time to introduce paper.

The student's first actual cutting is in short random snips. There is no forward or lateral direction to cutting at this stage.

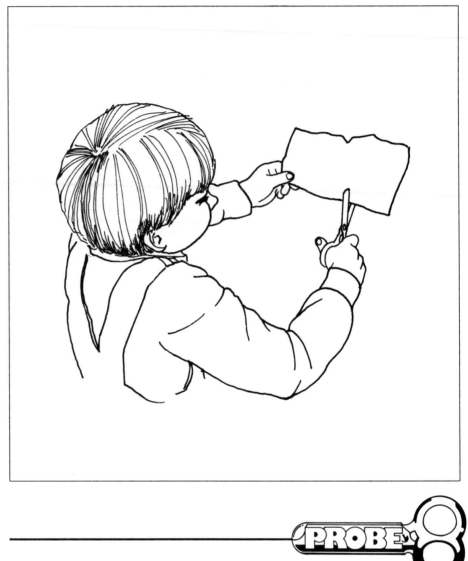

PROBE

What are the first four stages of scissor skill development?

Describe the type of cutting in which the scissors and paper are in actual contact for the first time.

Stage 5   The student manipulates scissors in a forward motion.

The first direction in which the beginning scissor user can manipulate the scissors is forward. The student begins to learn to aim the scissors at a forward visual goal, such as the other side of the paper. This is no longer random cutting; it is cutting to get to the edge of the paper or to make smaller pieces of paper.

At this stage, often it is difficult for the beginner to use standard paper. To help the student succeed in directing the beginning snips forward across the paper, try providing heavier paper, such as index cards, construction paper, oaktag, envelopes, or postcards. These heavier papers are more likely to remain firm between the scissor blades instead of bending or ripping midtask.

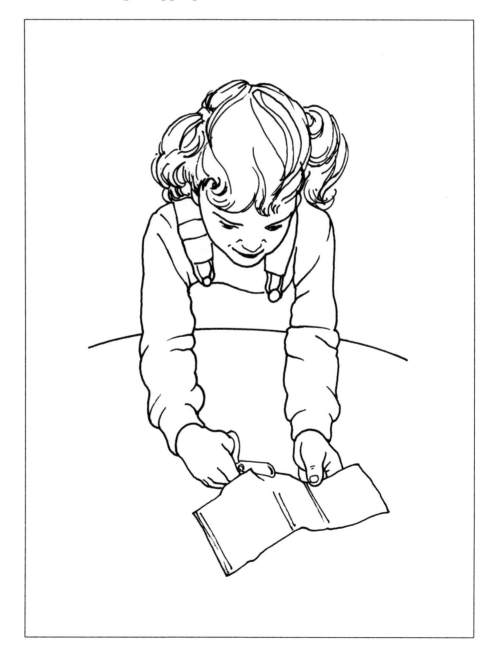

With practice, the beginning scissor user will be able to manipulate the scissors to cut across a one-inch strip of paper in any fashion, then across a four-inch strip, and then across six- and eight-inch strips.

Basically, the student's goal is merely to get across the paper, and it is not necessary to complicate the task by trying to keep the scissors on a cutting line. By increasing the width of the papers gradually, the teacher builds success into the program.

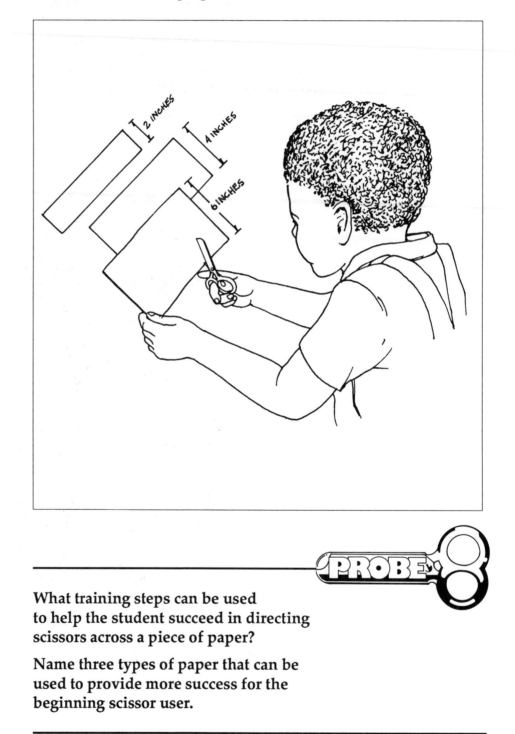

What training steps can be used to help the student succeed in directing scissors across a piece of paper?

Name three types of paper that can be used to provide more success for the beginning scissor user.

Stage 6   The student coordinates the lateral direction of scissors.

After learning to manipulate the scissors in a forward direction and consistently cut across paper in any fashion, the student is ready to begin coordinating the lateral movements of the scissors to stay on or within lines.

To remain successful at this stage, the student may need to practice cutting inside thick lines. Have the student cut within a six-inch line at first. Gradually decrease the width, offering opportunities to cut within a four-inch line, within a two-inch line, and then within a one-inch line.

To keep the student succeeding throughout the tasks, we must be careful to expect only one new skill performance at a time. The student practices snipping motions at first, without complicating the task with control of the paper. Then the student practices directing the snips across a piece of paper without attempting to stay on a line. Throughout, it is important to provide all the assistance needed to ensure the student's success and continued motivation. In addition to verbal encouragement, this assistance can take the form of activity modification and scissor or paper adaptations.

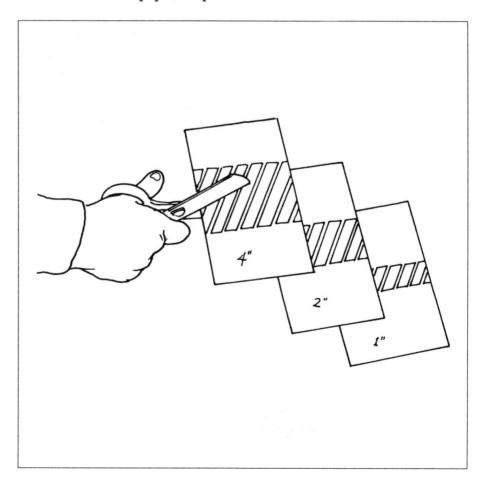

19

Refining Scissor Skills

The sequential scissor stages thus far have built a strong motoric foundation. The student has developed the prerequisites for refining the scissor skills.

Stage 7 The student cuts a straight forward line.

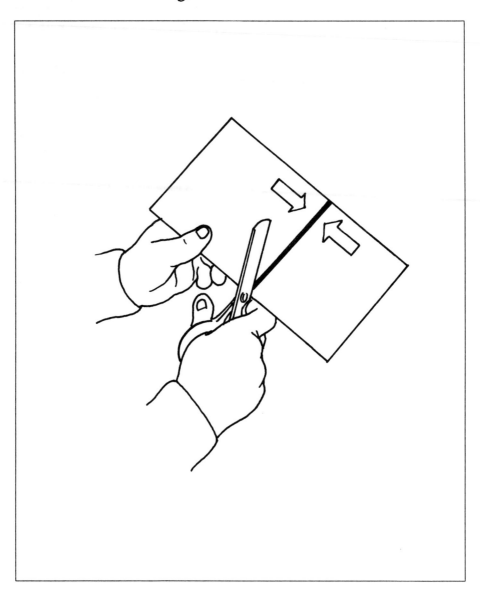

The beginner first learns to cut forward in a straight line. Draw thick, straight lines on paper, using a marking pen. Have the student practice cutting forward on those lines. Then draw thinner lines and have the student continue to practice cutting forward.

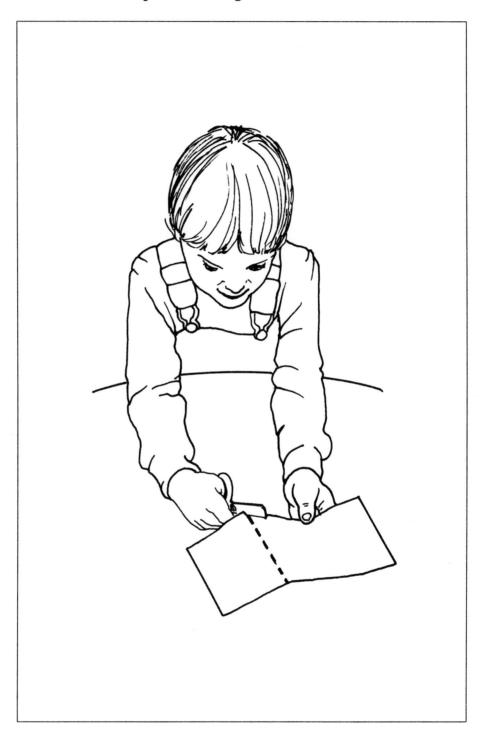

Stage 8 The student cuts simple geometric shapes.

Now the student is ready to practice cutting simple geometric shapes.

Cutting the square and the rectangle promotes scissor skill refinement because these shapes consist of straight lines, which the student has learned to cut already.

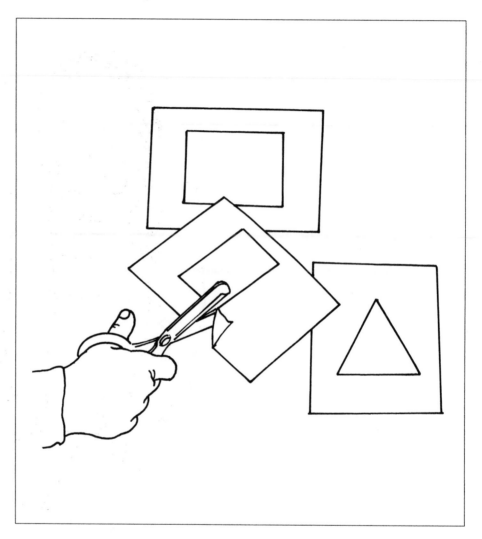

The triangle is the next line drawing the student cuts. It is made up of lines the student already knows how to cut, but they are at a new angle.

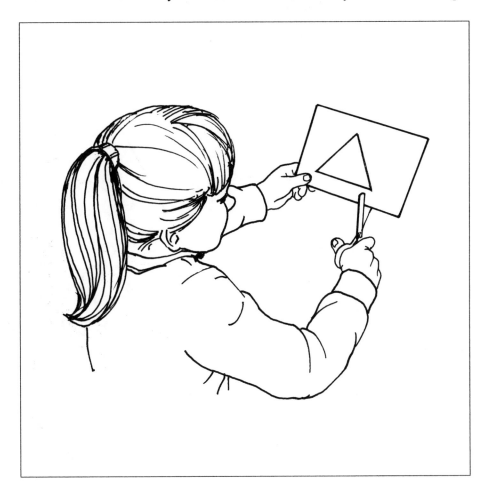

After learning to control the scissors to cut straight lines, the beginner practices cutting along curved lines. The semicircle is introduced, and then the circle.

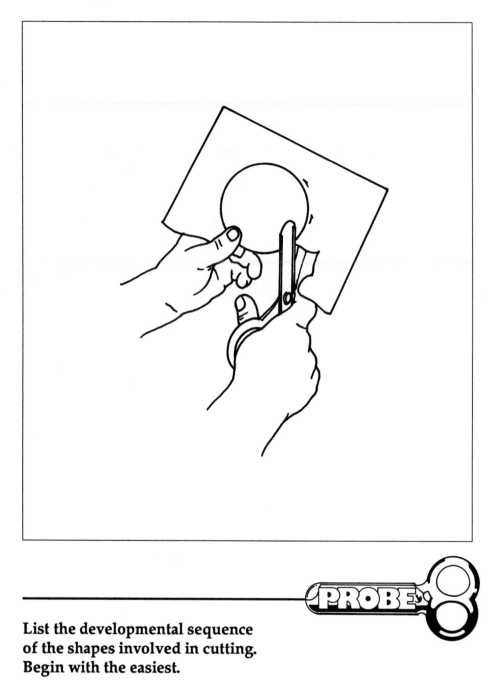

List the developmental sequence
of the shapes involved in cutting.
Begin with the easiest.

Stage 9 The student cuts simple figure shapes.

With practice, the student learns to refine the scissor action. Soon the student can cut out simple shapes with accuracy.

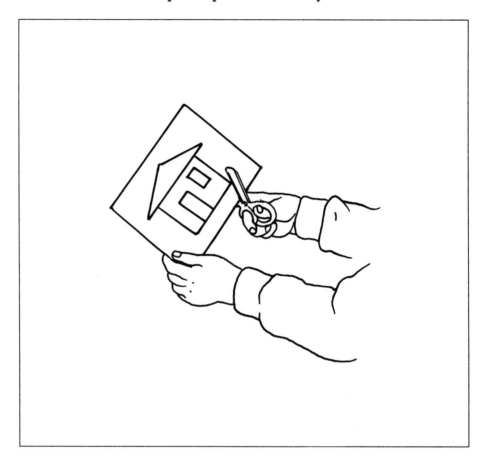

At first the task is to keep the scissors straight and turn the paper when a curve or direction change is necessary. Gradually the student learns to hold the paper still with the assisting hand while turning the scissors with the lead hand. The initial attempts to do this may be awkward, but with practice the movement becomes coordinated and smooth.

Stage 10 The student cuts complex figure shapes.

The student refines the ability to use two hands together for a task, and masters turning the paper or scissors to match line direction changes.

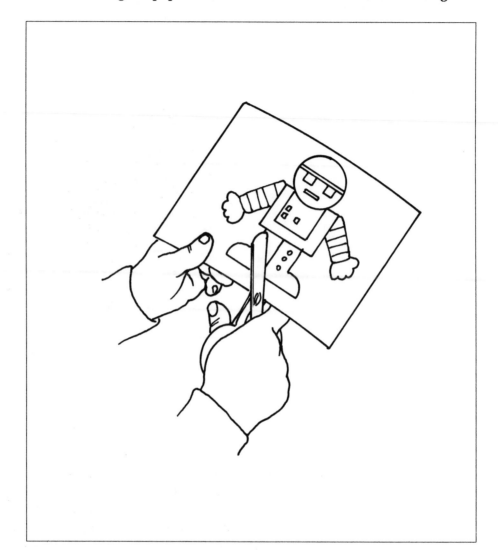

Stage 11 The student cuts nonpaper materials.

After learning to cut on regular papers, the student learns to adjust the scissor movements to cut different paper textures and weights. Then the student learns to cut string, tape, cloth, and other items.

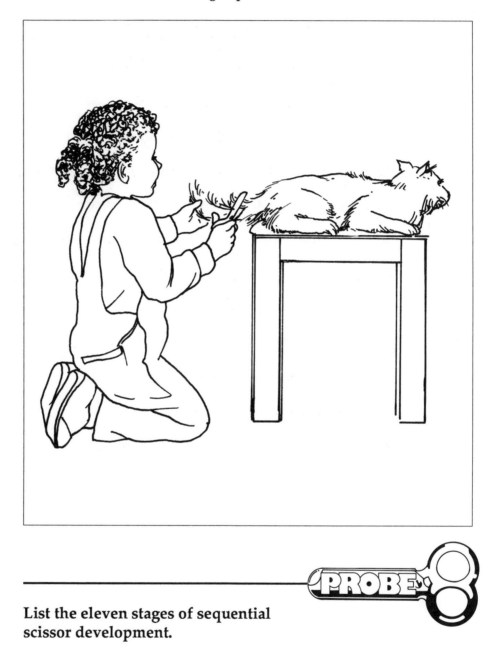

PROBE

List the eleven stages of sequential scissor development.

Overview of Developmental Stages in Acquiring Scissor Skills

Stage 1 The student shows an interest in scissors.

Stage 2 The student holds and manipulates scissors appropriately.

Stage 3 The student opens and closes scissors in a controlled fashion.

Stage 4 The student cuts short random snips.

Stage 5 The student manipulates scissors in a forward motion.

Stage 6 The student coordinates the lateral direction of scissors.

Stage 7 The student cuts a straight forward line.

Stage 8 The student cuts simple geometric shapes.

Stage 9 The student cuts simple figure shapes.

Stage 10 The student cuts complex figure shapes.

Stage 11 The student cuts nonpaper materials.

Checklist for Assessing Scissor Skills

Student's Name _____

Date of Assessment		Developmental Stage	Date Achieved
	1	Student shows an interest in scissors	
	2	Student holds and manipulates scissors appropriately	
	3	Student opens and closes scissors in a controlled fashion	
	4	Student cuts short random snips	
	5	Student manipulates scissors in a forward motion	
		Student cuts across a one-inch strip of paper in any fashion	
		Student cuts across a four-inch strip of paper in any fashion	
		Student cuts across a six-inch strip of paper in any fashion	
		Student cuts across an eight-inch strip of paper in any fashion	
	6	Student coordinates the lateral direction of scissors	
		Student cuts across paper, staying within a six-inch line	
		Student cuts across paper, staying within a four-inch line	
		Student cuts across paper, staying within a two-inch line	
		Student cuts across paper, staying within a one-inch line	
	7	Student cuts a straight forward line	
		Student cuts a thick line made with a marking pen	
		Student cuts a thinner line made with a marking pen	
	8	Student cuts simple geometric shapes	
		Student cuts out a square or rectangle	
		Student cuts out a triangle	
		Student cuts out a semicircle	
		Student cuts out a circle	
	9	Student cuts simple figure shapes	
	10	Student cuts complex figure shapes	
	11	Student cuts nonpaper materials	

Date _____

Comments _____

_____

_____

3 Choosing Appropriate Cutting Materials

A variety of textures and weights of materials can be used for cutting practice. While learning to manipulate scissors, some students are more apt to succeed with oaktag, index cards, construction paper, and other thicker papers. Later the student can refine the skills by cutting brown paper bags, standard paper, wax paper, aluminum foil, and onionskin paper.

When the student is ready to progress to nonpaper products, you can present string, tape, fabric, clay, flower stems, and other imaginative materials for the student to cut.

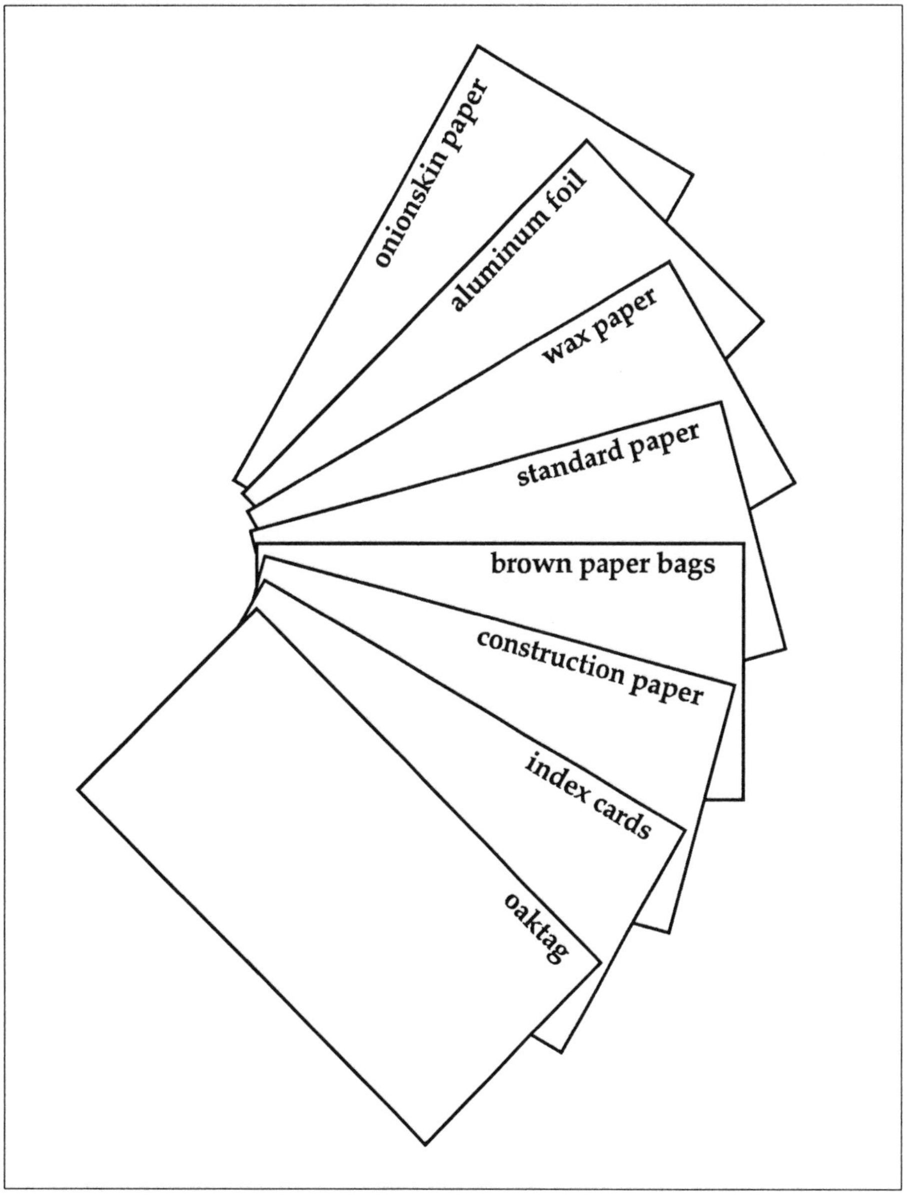

4 Pre-Scissor Experience Games

Eye-hand coordination is required for manipulating scissors. A number of games can be played in the classroom or at home to strengthen this important skill. A few games are described here, and some pages are left blank so you may record your own favorites.

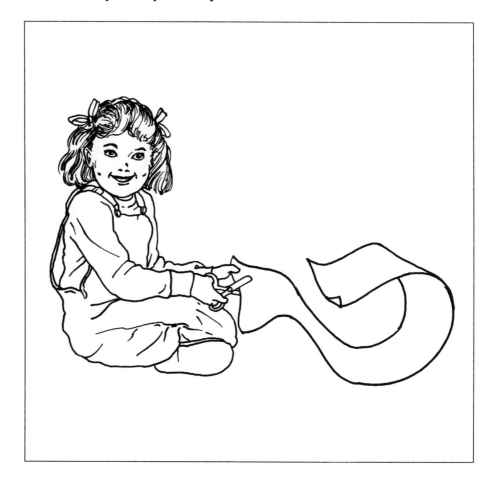

■ Pick-up Relay Games

Purpose To practice opening and closing tools like scissors

Scissor Skill Level Stage 3

Materials • Two buckets or other containers
• Salad servers, salad or bread tongs, or other tong-type tools
• Bells, aluminum foil balls, marshmallows, cotton balls, plastic toys, cookies, blocks, poker chips, yarn pom-poms, shelled peanuts, and other objects

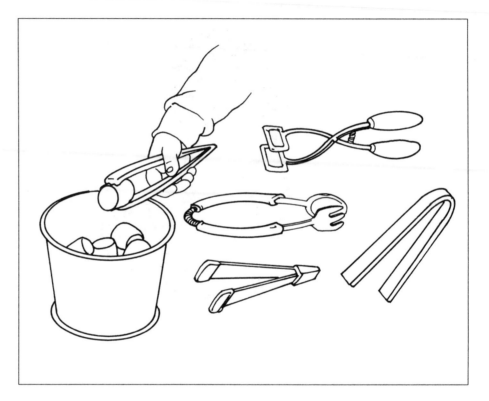

The Game Fill one bucket with objects. Have students use a tool to pick up an object from one bucket, run across the room, and drop it in the other bucket.

Variations Place the objects in boxes of sand or buckets of colored, soapy, or scented water.

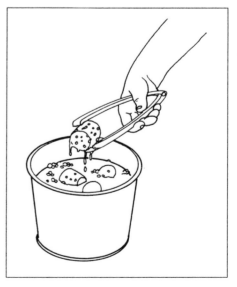

■ Squeeze Play

Purpose To practice opening and closing hands

Scissor Skill Level Stage 3

Materials
- Squirt guns, turkey basters or other bulb squeezers
- Water
- Balloons, whipped cream, body paints, soap suds in a pan

Five Games
1. See who has "the quickest draw" with squirt guns.

2. Hang balloons from the ceiling with string. Let the children make them move by shooting them with squirt guns.

3. Have children use squirt guns or bulb squeezers to spray balloons that have whipped cream faces drawn on them.

4. Let students use squirt guns or bulb squeezers to wash body paints off their own or other children's hands or feet.

5. Have students squirt water into a pan of soap suds to make more bubbles.

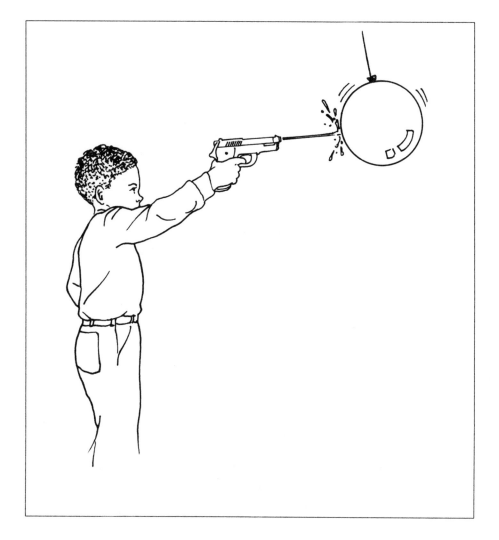

■ Paper Punch Games

Purpose To practice directing a tool in a forward motion

Scissor Skill Level Stages 3, 4, 5

Materials
- Paper punch
- Stiff paper or index cards
- Laces
- Crayons or marking pens

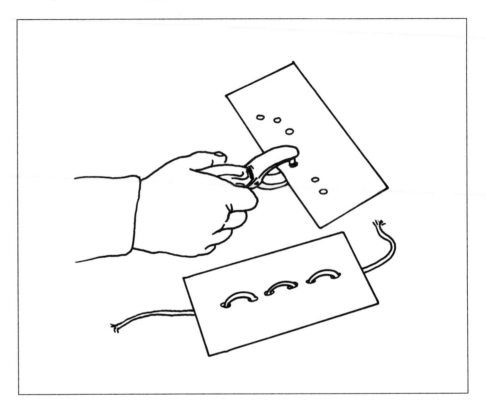

Three Games

1. Have the student use the paper punch to make random holes in stiff paper. Then the student can lace the card or connect the holes with crayon lines.

2. Draw colored dots or small circles on paper or an index card. Have the student use the tool to punch out the colored pattern.

3. Write CANDY STORE at the top of a piece of stiff paper. Draw a path from the bottom of the paper to the Candy Store. Have the student punch holes along the path to the destination.

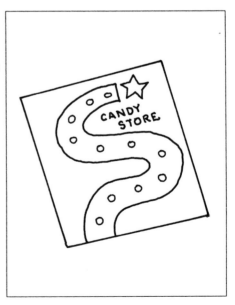

Pre-Scissor Experience Games

Purpose _____

_____

_____

Scissor Skill Level _____

_____

Materials _____

_____

_____

_____

Games _____

_____

_____

_____

_____

_____

_____

_____

_____

_____

_____

_____

_____

_____

_____

Pre-Scissor Experience Games

Purpose _____

_____

_____

Scissor Skill Level _____

_____

Materials _____

_____

_____

_____

Games _____

_____

_____

_____

_____

_____

_____

_____

_____

_____

_____

_____

_____

_____

_____

_____

_____

5 Types of Scissors Available

Selecting Scissors

The scissors you choose for a student should be designed to offer maximum success for that individual. Consider these factors:

Handedness — Is the student right- or left-handed?

Hand Size — Is the student a child or an adult?

Motor Coordination — Does the student have any physical disabilities or limitations which require adaptive scissors?

Trainer Assistance — Will the scissors permit the type of trainer assistance needed to ensure student success?

Purchase Information

The products described here are available from a number of distributors. The outlets and addresses listed here are included for your convenience only.

■ Electric Scissors

Handedness The student can be right- or left-handed.

Hand Size For children or adults

Motor Coordination The student does not need to be able to open and close the hand or isolate movement of the index and middle fingers and thumb.

Trainer Assistance Electric scissors are large enough for both the student and trainer to hold simultaneously.

Purchase Information These are available in any department or sewing store.

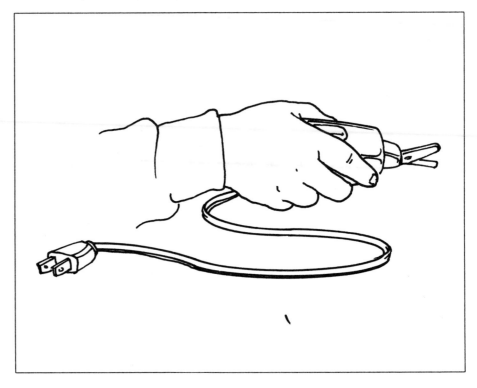

■ Nonloop (Easy-Grip) Scissors

These scissors have become more and more popular. They are excellent to use in teaching the beginning or older scissor user who has physical disabilities that make finger isolation difficult.

Handedness — These can be purchased for right- or left-handed use.

Hand Size — For children or adults

Additional Feature — These scissors can be purchased with pointed or rounded tips.

Motor Coordination — The student must be able to open and close the hand but needs no refined index and middle finger and thumb isolation.

Trainer Assistance — Often, only minimal trainer assistance is needed. The trainer can hold the back end of the scissors while the student squeezes the middle. The student can rest the wrist on the table while cutting, reducing the need for controlled wrist stability.

Purchase Information — Developmental Learning Materials, 7440 Natchez Ave., Niles, IL 60648

Fred Sammons, Inc., Box 32, Brookfield, IL 60513-0032

Lakeshore Curriculum Materials, 2695 E. Dominguez St., P.O. Box 6261, Carson, CA 90749

Teaching Resources, 100 Boylston St., Boston, MA 02116

Childcraft Educational Corp., 20 Kilmer Road, P.O. Box 3081, Edison, NJ 08818-3081

Teaching Tools/Little Red Schoolhouse, 3154 N. 34th St., Phoenix, AZ 85017

■ Safety Scissors

With these safety scissors, trainers can be more confident that fingers will not be hurt while young hands are practicing cutting. The scissors are small in size and are appropriate for beginner scissor users.

Handedness   The student can be right- or left-handed.

Hand Size   For children

Motor Coordination   The student must be able to open and close the hand and isolate movement of the index and middle fingers and thumb.

Purchase Information   These scissors are available under various names in a variety of small sizes and shapes, all with safety blades. They can be purchased in toy or children's shops, or by mail from the following:

Sure-Cut Safety Scissors, Lakeshore Curriculum Materials, 2695 E. Dominguez St., P.O. Box 6261, Carson, CA 90749

ChildSafe Scissors, Constructive Playthings, 1227 E. 119th St., Grandview, MO 64030

Superscissors, Childcraft Educational Corp., 20 Kilmer Road, P.O. Box 3081, Edison, NJ 08818-3081

Super Safety Scissors, Teaching Tools/Little Red Schoolhouse, 3154 N. 34th St., Phoenix, AZ 85017

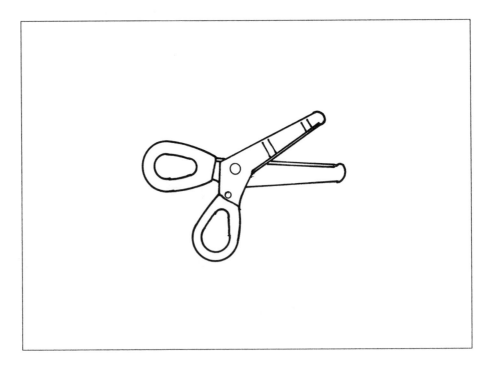

■ Easy-Cut Plastic Scissors

These scissors have no blades or metal on the blade that could accidentally cut a child. They won't become dull because they are made of tempered polycarbonate, similar to ceramic.

Handedness These scissors are for either right- or left-handed use.

Hand Size For children

Motor Coordination The student must be able to open and close the hand and isolate the movement of the index and middle fingers and thumb.

Purchase Information These scissors are available under various names and are made by several manufacturers. They can be purchased in children's shops and in the school supply section of department stores, or by mail from:

Lakeshore Curriculum Materials, 2695 E. Dominguez St., P.O. Box 6261, Carson, CA 90749

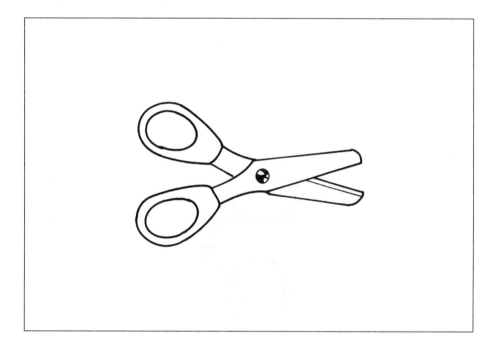

■ Cushion-Grip Scissors

Soft vinyl-cushioned handles provide easy-to-hold loops for beginning scissor users. They can be purchased with pointed or blunt ends.

Handedness Can be purchased for right- or left-handed use.

Hand Size For children

Motor Coordination The student must be able to open and close the hand and isolate the movement of the index and middle fingers and thumb.

Purchase Information These scissors are available under various names in most children's shops and school supply sections of department stores, or they can be ordered from:

Lakeshore Curriculum Materials, 2695 E. Dominguez St., P.O. Box 6261, Carson, CA 90749

Childcraft Educational Corp., 20 Kilmer Road, P.O. Box 3081, Edison, NJ 08818-3081

Teaching Tools/Little Red Schoolhouse, 3154 N. 34th St., Phoenix, AZ 85017

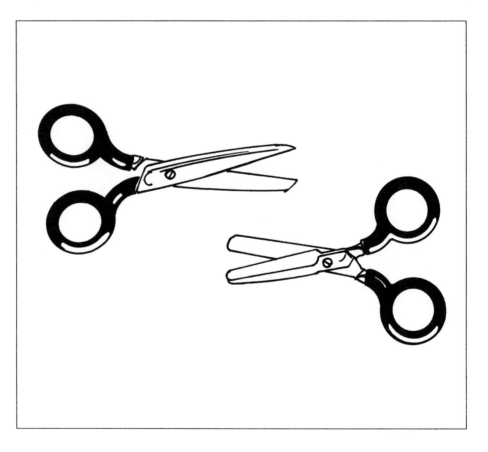

■ Decorator Scissors

These child-sized scissors are made in a variety of animal, vehicle, or other play shapes. They are brightly colored and highly motivating for children.

Handednesss   Can be used for right- or left-handed cutting.

Hand Size   For children

Motor Coordination   The student must be able to open and close the hand and isolate the movement of the index and middle fingers and thumb.

Purchase Information   These scissors are available in most department, school supply, and toy stores.

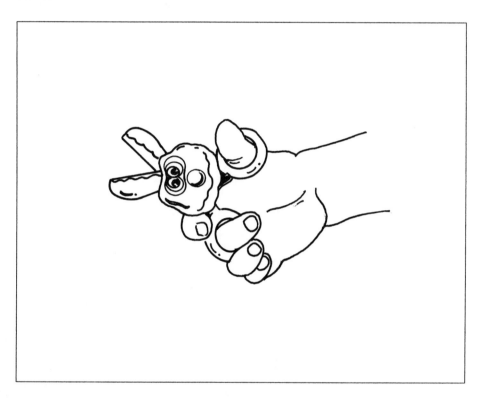

■ Double-Ring Training Scissors

Handedness Can be purchased for right- or left-handed use.

Hand Size For children

Motor Coordination The student must be able to open and close the hand and isolate movement of the index and middle fingers and thumb.

Trainer Assistance Double-ring scissors are ideal for beginning scissor users who need help in initiating the task. The trainer places a hand over the child's scissor grasp and guides the student to success. Gradually, trainer assistance is faded.

Purchase Information Childcraft Corp., 20 Kilmer Road, P.O. Box 3081, Edison, NJ 08818-3081

Constructive Playthings, 11100 Harry Hines Blvd., Dallas, TX 75229

Developmental Learning Materials, 7440 Natchez Ave., Niles, IL 60648

Lakeshore Curriculum Materials, 2695 E. Dominguez St., P.O. Box 6261, Carson, CA 90749

Nasco Learning Fun, 1524 Princeton Ave., Modesto, CA 95352

Teaching Tools/Little Red Schoolhouse, 3154 N. 34th St., Phoenix, AZ 85017

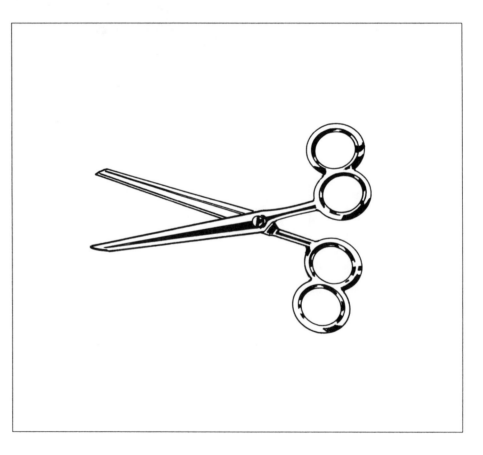

■ Double-Loop Training Scissors

Handedness	Can be purchased for right- or left-handed use.
Hand Size	For adults or older children
Motor Coordination	The student must be able to open and close the hand and isolate movement of the index and middle fingers and thumb.
Trainer Assistance	Dual-loop scissors are ideal for teaching scissor usage to older students. The trainer can hold the end loops and help guide the beginning cutting attempts. Assistance can be faded gradually as the student gains more control. These scissors also can be used for children who tend to be tactilely defensive or who have a difficult time tolerating being touched (as in the hand-over-hand touch of the double-ring training scissors).
Purchase Information	Double-loop scissors are available through most medical equipment distributors or teaching supply stores, or by mail from:

J.A. Preston Corp., 71 Fifth Avenue, New York, NY 10003

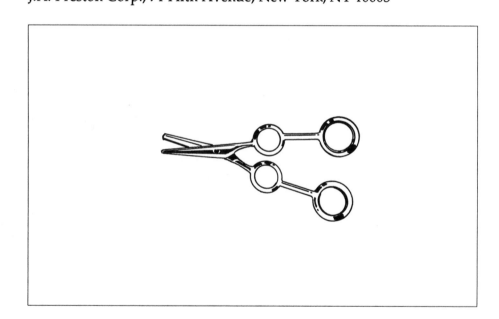

■ Adult Scissors

Handedness   Can be purchased for right- or left-handed use.

Hand Size   For adults

Motor Coordination   The student must be able to open and close the hand and isolate movements of the index, middle, and ring fingers and thumb.

Trainer Assistance   The student should require minimal, if any, trainer assistance.

Purchase Information   These scissors can be purchased in a variety of department, school supply, and sewing stores, or by mail from:

Teaching Tools/Little Red Schoolhouse, 3154 N. 34th St., Phoenix, AZ 85017

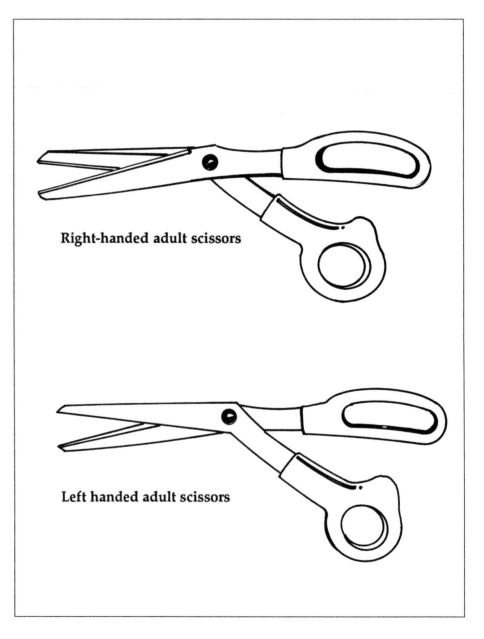

Right-handed adult scissors

Left handed adult scissors

■ Three-Hole Scissors

Handedness Can be purchased for right- or left-handed use.

Hand Size For adults

Motor Coordination The student must be able to open and close the hand and isolate the movement of index and middle fingers and thumb.

Trainer Assistance The student should require minimal, if any, trainer assistance.

Purchase Information Three-hole scissors are available through most medical equipment distributors or teaching supply stores, or by mail from:

A. Daigger & Co., Educational Teaching Aids Division, 159 W. Kinzie St., Chicago, IL 60610

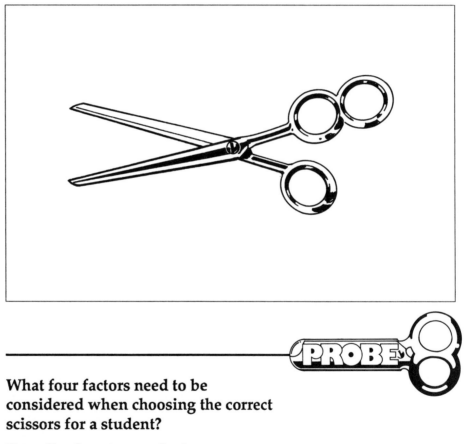

PROBE

What four factors need to be considered when choosing the correct scissors for a student?

Describe four types of scissors.

49

6 Adaptations in Scissor Instruction

Prerequisites for scissor usage were explained earlier. Teachers often ask if a student can be taught scissor skills if any of these precursor skills are missing. Each situation needs to be reviewed individually. However, when students are having difficulties in specific areas, certain adaptive techniques can be useful.

Problem Area:
Balance

We determined earlier that balance is absolutely essential as a prerequisite for cutting. If the student's balance is off, all attention goes toward worry about falling. If the student's trunk is leaning to the side or in constant motion, it provides a poor basis of support from which to control the more refined movements necessary for cutting.

Be sure the child is sitting in a stable chair. Feet should be touching the floor. If the only available chairs are too high, use a box or stepstool under the student's feet. If the student is in a wheelchair, be sure the footrests fit and are being used. Some students may have better balance in an armchair or with pillow support on either side. With this type of secure base, the student can focus attention on the task at hand.

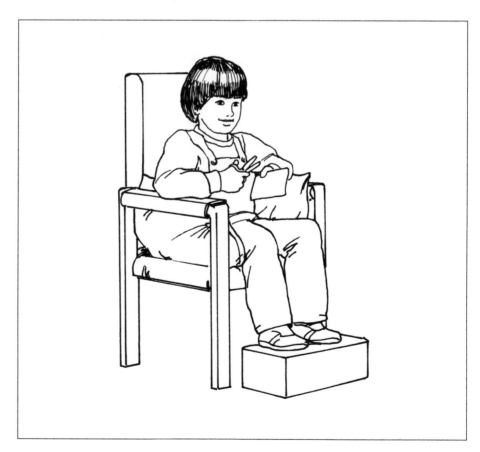

Problem Area:
Stability

Control and stability develop from a proximal-to-distal direction. The student is now sitting in a balanced position, so there is a stable base. There must be stability at the shoulder for the elbow to work, stability at the elbow for the wrist to work, stability at the wrist for the hand to work, and stability on one side of the hand for the other side to use scissors to cut.

Sitting firmly in an overstuffed chair can give support at the shoulders. This can have the effect of helping the student rest the arms on the trunk. With upper arms on the trunk, the lower arms are free to bend at the elbow and cut.

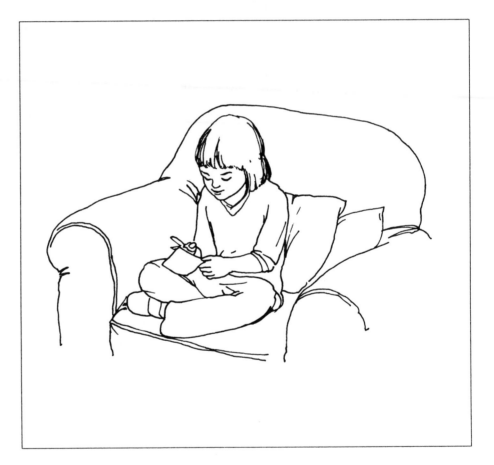

The desk or table can be a source of stability. Let the student lean forward with one or both elbows resting on the flat surface. This provides stability at the elbows and shoulders and allows freedom at the forearms and hands.

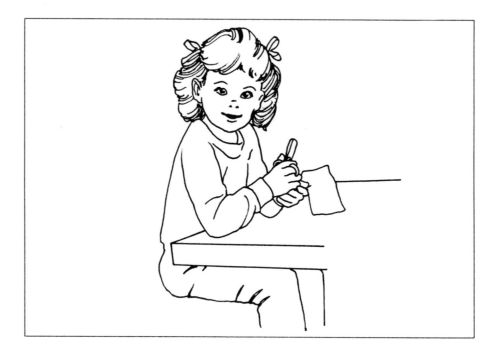

For variation, have the student rest the entire forearm on the table. This provides stability above the wrist and allows the scissor user to achieve maximum wrist and hand control.

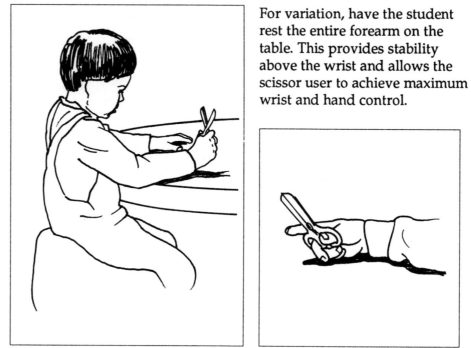

If the student needs additional assistance to separate one side of the hand from the other, leaning the radial (little finger) side of the scissor hand on the table may be what is needed. This stabilizes the radial side so the other side is free to open and close for cutting.

Problem Area:
Grasp and Release

Grasping and releasing are very important to scissor usage. Usually it is considered unlikely that a student will cut if unable to grasp. One option, however, is for this student to use electric scissors. These require the student merely to push a button to make them work.

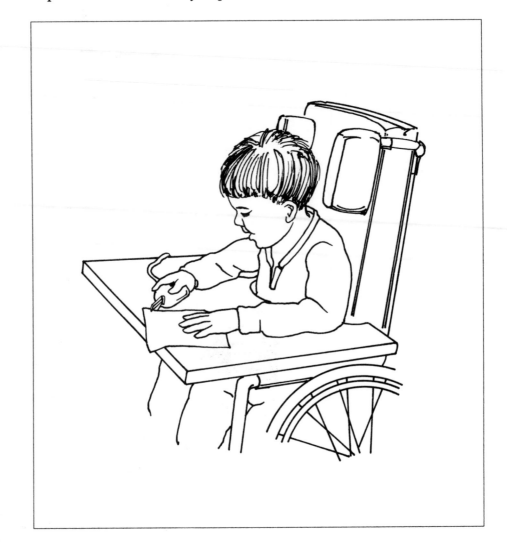

If the student has some grasp but it is unrefined, nonloop scissors may provide success. These scissors close when they are squeezed with a whole hand grasp. No finger isolation is needed. They open with a spring action when the hand is relaxed. No specific opening motion is necessary.

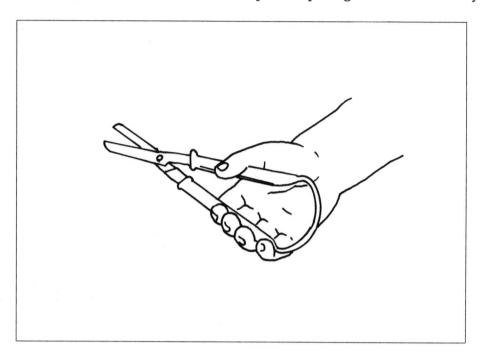

Another way to provide assistance is to help the student experience the action of opening and closing the scissors. Double-loop scissors allow you to hold the back loops and manipulate the blades while the student feels the action. Gradually, assistance can fade as the student takes over the task.

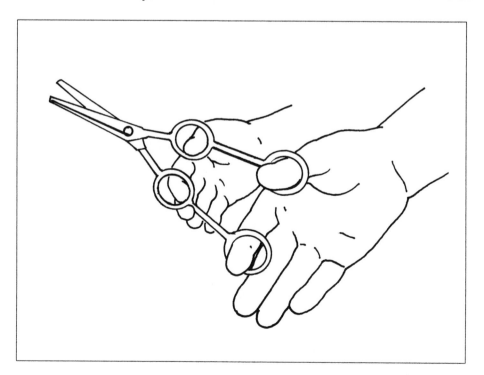

Problem Area:
Poor Two-Hand Usage

Some students have trouble using both hands in a lead-assist fashion.
Others may be able to use only one side of the body. To begin the
scissor concepts, try holding the paper so the student can concentrate
attention on the scissor hand.

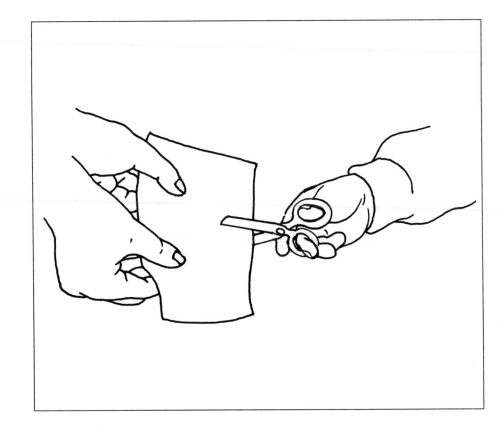

Try taping the paper to the edge of the table. Then the student can cut without having to hold the paper.

Many hemiplegic, or one-sided, students can use their involved side to assist. With practice and encouragement, often they can lean their involved side against the paper to hold it on the table. By shifting their weight and moving the paper with their elbow and forearm, they can manage some basic cutting skills.

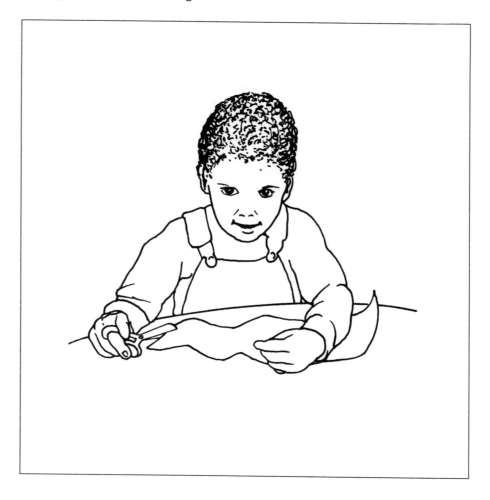

Problem Area: Finger Isolation

Nonloop scissors do not require finger isolation. Electric scissors also can be a choice for students who have difficulty in this area.

Problem Area: Bending and Tearing Paper

Students who have limited experience with cutting often have the problem of paper getting caught in the scissors and then bending or tearing. The problem is created because these students are cutting completely through the paper at each cut and doing so without adequate lateral stability. They need to use shorter, more controlled cutting movements. This can be achieved by binding the handles of the scissors or binding the section where the scissor blades cross. Or try using heavy paper, which may provide just the right amount of resistance needed for extra stability.

To bind the handle loops, use string, tape, or yarn. This prevents the scissors from completely shutting and allows for more continuous contact.

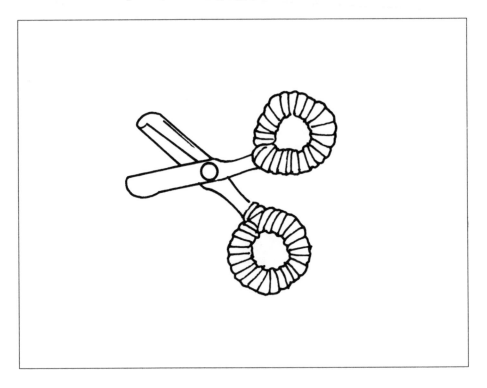

To bind the crossed-blade section, twist a rubber band around it several times. This provides resistance when the blades are opened and draws the student's attention to the closing process.

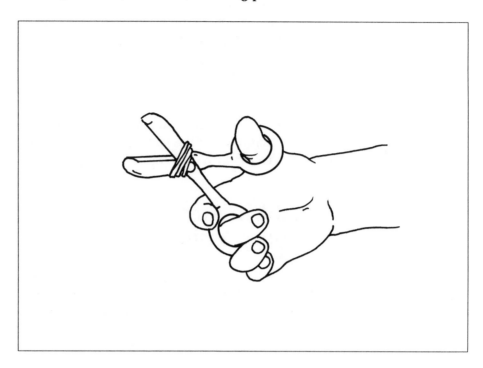

Problem Area:
Opening the Scissors

Some students have difficulty controlling the opening of the scissors. Try using nonloop scissors, which are designed to open automatically with a spring action.

Problem Area:
Closing the Scissors

For students who have difficulty squeezing the scissors, bind the crossed-blade section with a rubber band as described above. The band contracts and pulls the blades together, thus requiring little force on the student's part.

Problem Area:
Shaking Movements

Students who have intention tremors, mild athetosis, or other types of physical disabilities may need extra assistance with stabilization to control their shaky movements. Try using a weighted wrist cuff on the scissors hand. A cuff may or may not be necessary on the assisting paper-holding hand.

You may want to build a control pole. The pole is secured to a piece of wood that rests on the table. The whole unit can be attached to the table with Velcro® or a C-clamp, if necessary.

Problem Area:
Limited Vision

Students with limited vision may need extra cues to help them succeed at cutting. Use bright colors to draw the cutting lines, or use colors that provide a sharp contrast to the paper. Holes punched along the cutting lines will provide an extra tactile cue. String, yarn, or sandpaper can be used as template guides for cutting.

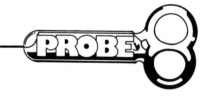

Name ten problem areas that may require adaptations.

What are the recommendations for each problem?

Velcro® is a registered trademark of Velcro U.S.A., Inc., Manchester, NH.

7 Classroom Scissor Activities

The following are a few classroom activities that can help the beginning scissor user improve coordination and direction. Blank activity sheets are provided for you to use in recording your own ideas.

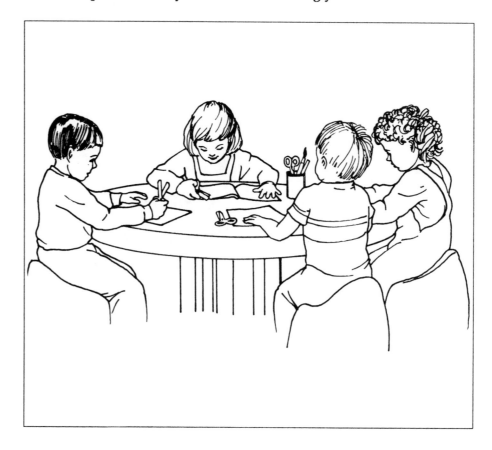

■ Classroom Scissor Activity

Purpose To practice directing the scissors

Scissor Skill Level Stages 5, 6, 7

Materials Paper punch
Paper
Scissors

Procedure Punch a hole or cluster of holes at the top and bottom of a sheet of paper. Have the student cut from one hole toward the other holes.

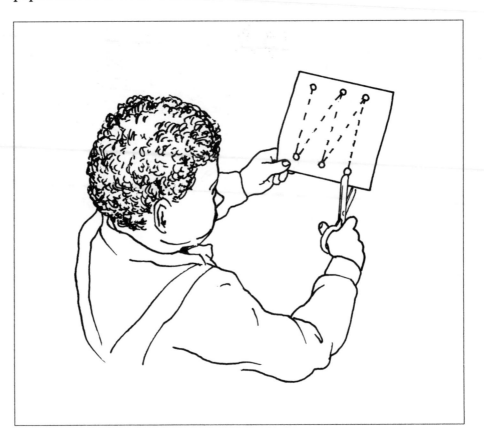

Cut from Hole to Hole

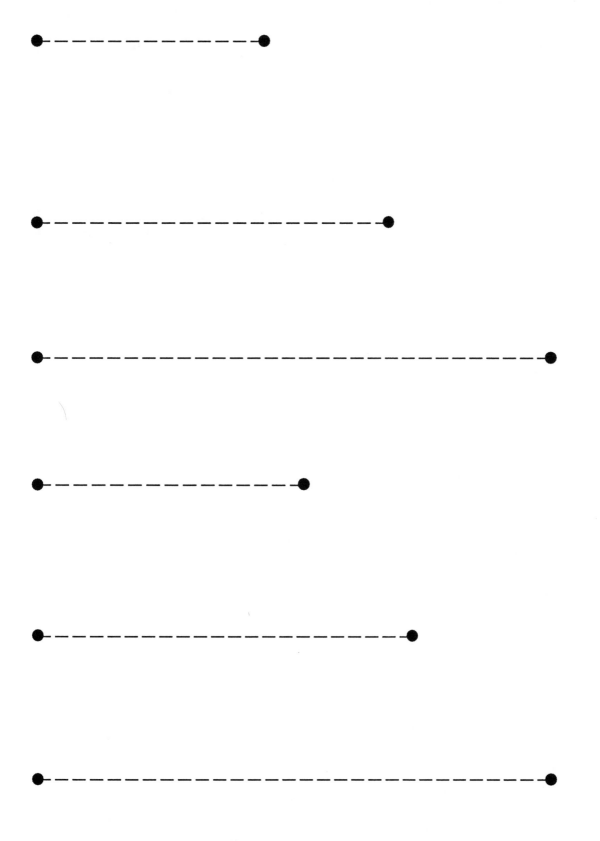

Cut from Hole to Hole

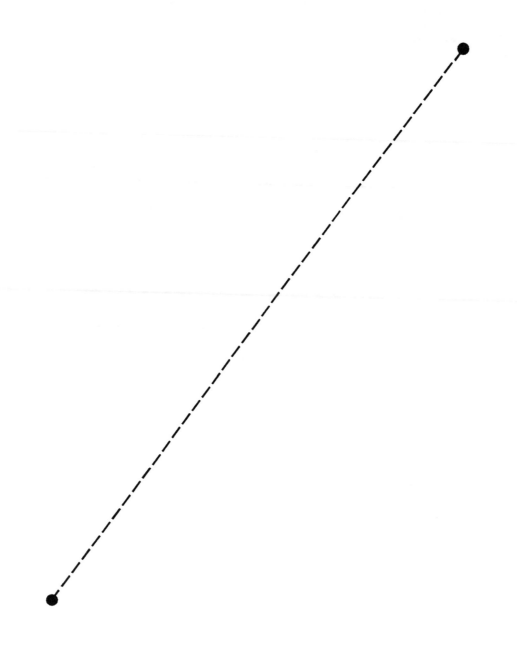

■ Classroom Scissor Activity

Purpose To practice directing the scissors

Scissor Skill Level Stages 5, 6, 7

Materials 3" X 5" index cards
Paper
Scissors
Glue
"Spot" materials (pieces of yarn, sandpaper, colored stickers, circles of tape, pieces of colored construction paper)

Procedure Randomly glue pieces or strips of spot materials on index cards. Have the student direct the scissors toward the spot and cut from spot to spot.

Later, glue the spot materials on sheets of paper, and have the student cut from spot to spot.

The larger the spot or strip, the better chance the student has for success. The more spots on the page, the more complex the task becomes.

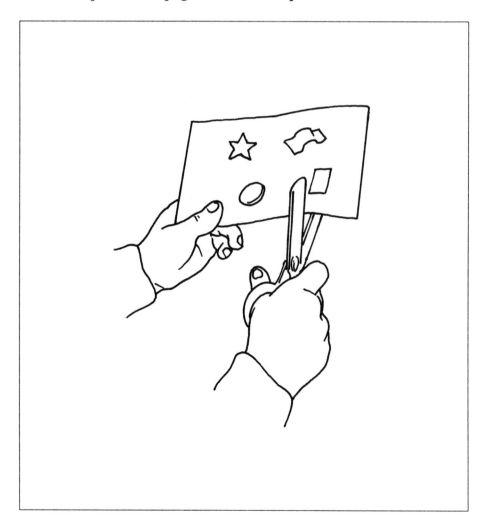

■ Classroom Scissor Activity

Purpose To practice directing the scissors

Scissor Skill Level Stages 5, 6, 7

Materials Paper
Scissors
Gumdrops, small marshmallows, or other sticky candies

Procedure Cut a gumdrop in half so it will stick to the designated spot. Have the student cut the paper in the direction of the gumdrop. When the gumdrop is reached, the student can eat it.

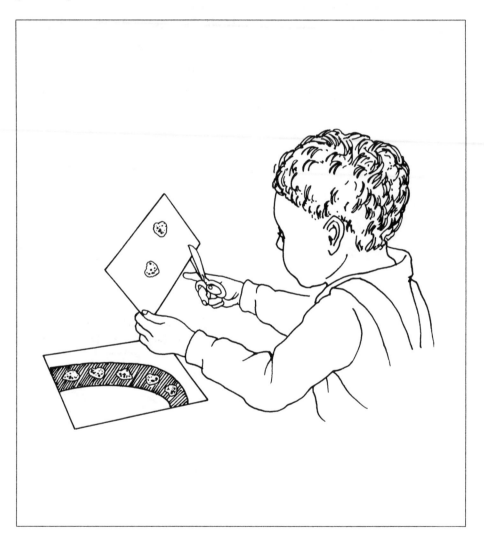

■ Classroom Scissor Activity

Purpose   To teach the student to control the direction of the scissors (cutting lines)

Scissor Skill Level   Stages 6, 7

Materials   Cardboard and craft knife (or wood and jigsaw)
Tape (or glue)
Paper strips
Scissors

Procedure   Make troughs in two pieces of cardboard or wood. Place paper between the pieces. Have the student cut the paper, using the troughs to help guide the scissors.

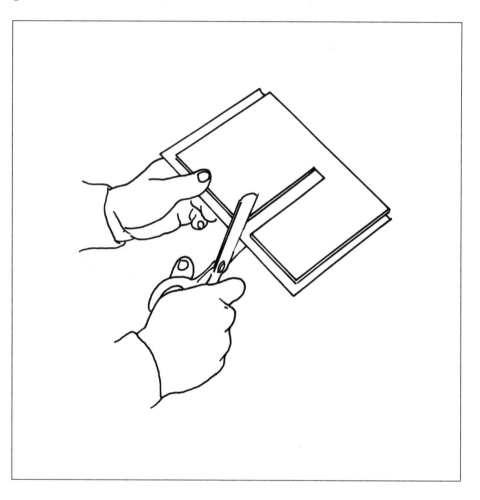

■ Classroom Scissor Activity

Purpose To teach the student to control the direction of the scissors (cutting lines)

Scissor Skill Level Stages 6, 7

Materials Stiff paper
Glue
Craft sticks
Scissors

Procedure Glue craft sticks parallel on a sheet of stiff paper. Have the student cut the paper between the sticks.

Initially, glue the sticks four to six inches apart. As coordination increases, glue them closer together.

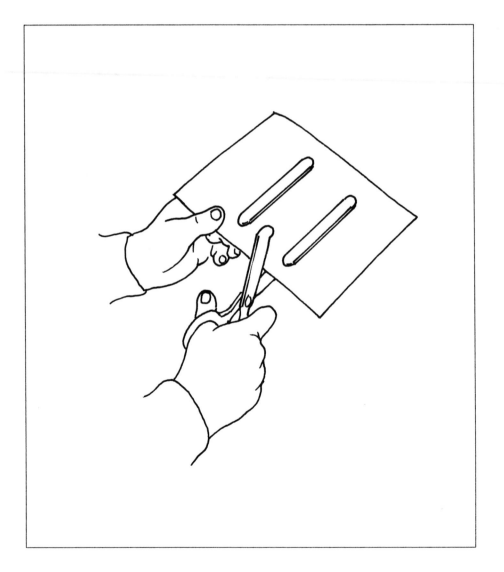

Variation Glue two pieces of yarn parallel. Have the student cut between the yarn strips.

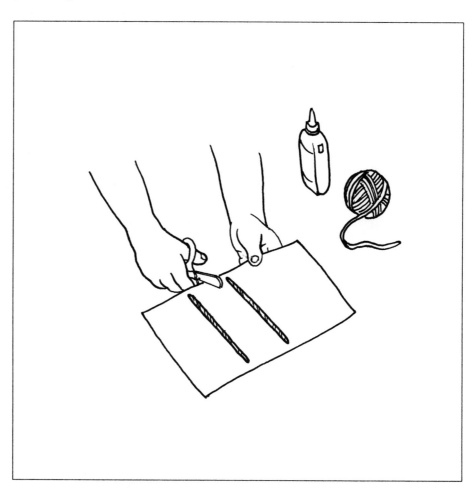

■ Classroom Scissor Activity

Purpose To teach the student to control the direction of the scissors (cutting lines)

Scissor Skill Level Stages 6, 7

Materials Construction paper
Sandpaper
Glue
Scissors

Procedure Glue two pieces of sandpaper parallel on a sheet of construction paper. Have the student cut the "line" between the sandpaper strips. The sandpaper texture serves as a cue if the student goes off the line.

Initially, place the sandpaper strips far apart. Move them closer to make a thinner "line" as the student gains confidence.

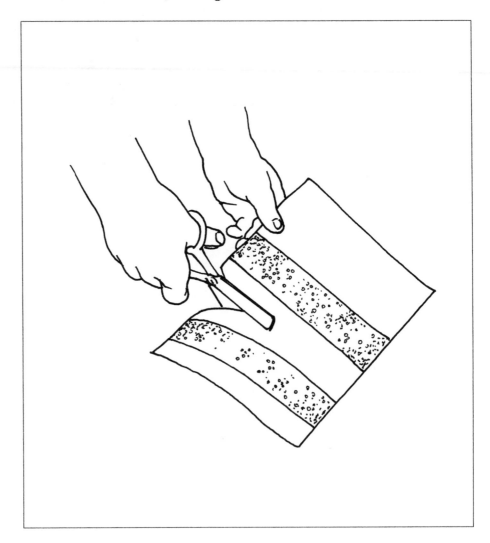

■ Classroom Scissor Activity

Purpose To teach the student to control the direction of the scissors (cutting lines)

Scissor Skill Level Stage 7

Materials Construction paper
Marking pens, paint, or crayons
Glue (optional)
Scissors

Procedure Draw or color one to six one-inch strips across the construction paper. Have the student cut within or on the colored areas.

Variation Cut one-inch strips from construction paper. Glue strips on a full sheet of construction paper. Have the student cut within or between the strips.

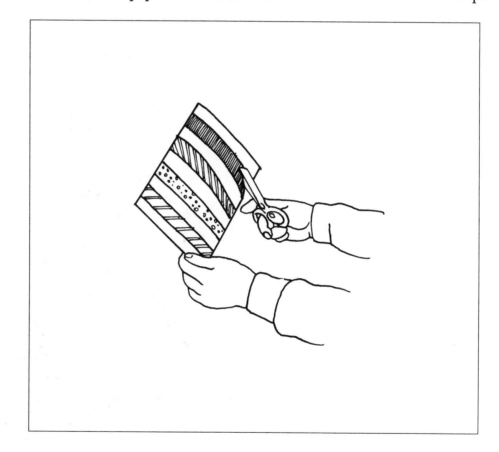

■ Classroom Scissor Activity

Purpose To teach the student to cut lines

Scissor Skill Level Stages 5, 6, 7

Materials Construction paper
Glue
Scissors

Procedure Have the student cut strips of construction paper, then glue the strips into circles and make chains.

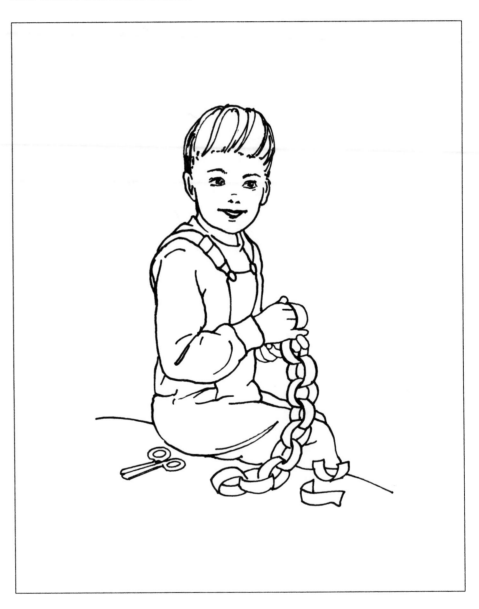

■ Classroom Scissor Activity

Purpose To teach the student to control the direction of the scissors (cutting diagonal lines)

Scissor Skill Level Stages 7, 8, 9

Materials Construction paper
Glue
Scissors
Marking pens (optional)

Procedure Cut strips of construction paper. Glue them diagonally across a sheet of paper. Have the student cut along the diagonal lines.

As coordination develops, use a larger sheet of paper and longer strips so the student has to cut a longer distance.

Variation Using colored marking pens, draw diagonal lines across paper. Have the student cut within or on the diagonal lines.

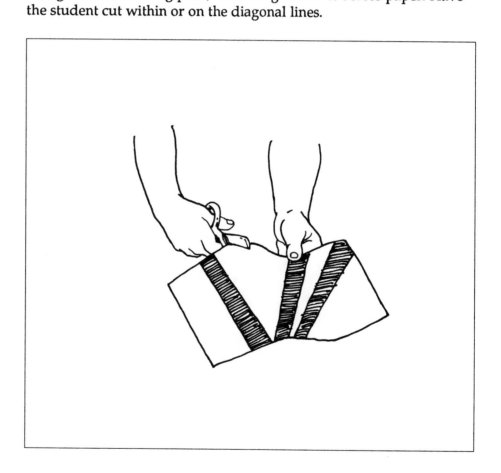

■ Classroom Scissor Activity

Purpose To teach the student to control the direction of the scissors (cutting lines)

Scissor Skill Level Stage 7

Materials Paper
Ruler
Pencil
Scissors

Procedure Draw a line across a sheet of paper. Cut strips up to the line, as shown. Fold alternate flaps up. Have the student cut along the flaps. The short cuts make it easier to get across the paper because it is done in small sections.

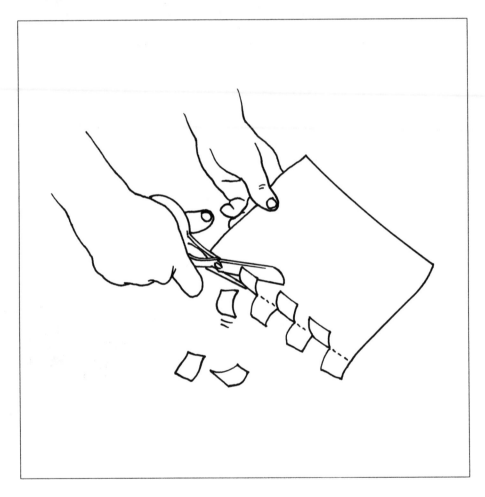

■ Classroom Scissor Activity

Purpose To teach the student to control the direction of the scissors (cutting lines)

Scissor Skill Level Stages 6, 7, 8, 9

Materials Paper
Paper punch
Scissors

Procedure Punch a line of holes along the edge of a piece of paper. Have the student cut off the strip along the hole-punched line.

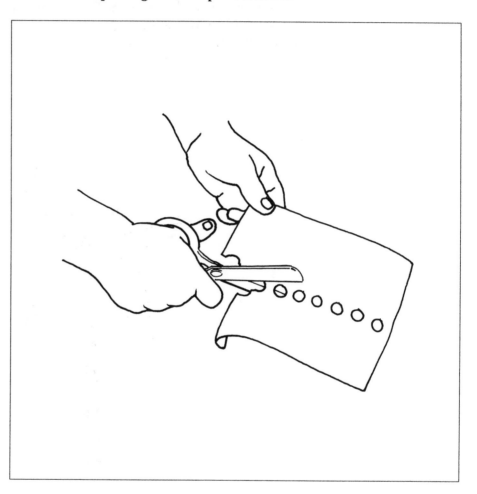

■ Classroom Scissor Activity

Purpose	To teach the student to control the direction of the scissors (cutting lines)
Scissor Skill Level	Stages 7, 8
Materials	Paper Pencil Scissors Pin Crayons
Procedure	Have the student color a pinwheel form, cut it out along the dotted lines, bring the left corners of each triangle to the middle, and fasten the pinwheel to the eraser of a pencil.

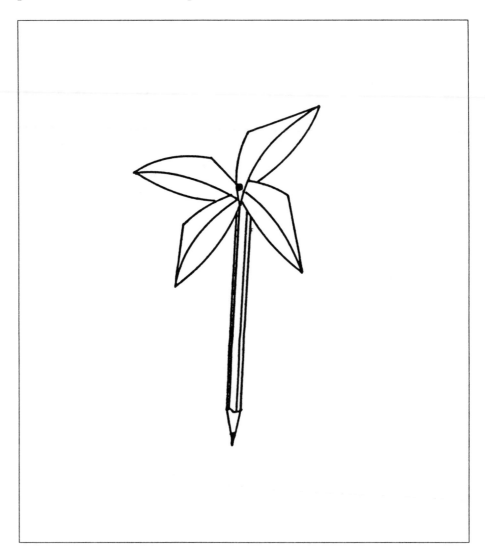

■ Classroom Scissor Activity

Purpose To teach the student to control the direction of the scissors (cutting curved lines)

Scissor Skill Level Stages 7, 8

Materials Two circular pieces of wood or cardboard
Paper
Scissors

Procedure Place a piece of paper between the two circles. Have the student cut out circles, using the wood or cardboard shape to guide the scissors in the curved direction.

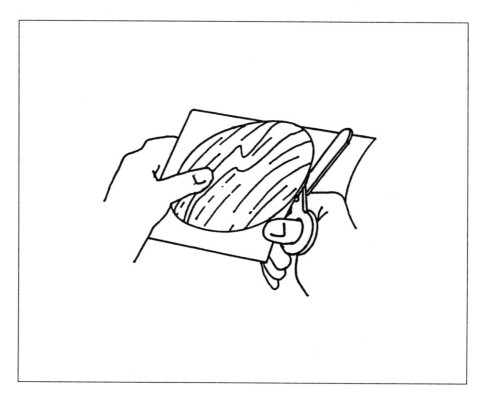

■ Classroom Scissor Activity

Purpose   To teach the student to control the direction of the scissors (cutting curved lines)

Scissor Skill Level   Stages 7, 8

Materials   Troughs in cardboard or wood
Tape or glue
Paper
Scissors

Procedure   Make troughs, as shown, in cardboard or wood. The troughs can vary from narrow to wide, depending on the student's skills. Tape or glue paper strips across the troughs. Have the student cut across the paper strips, using the troughs to guide the scissors.

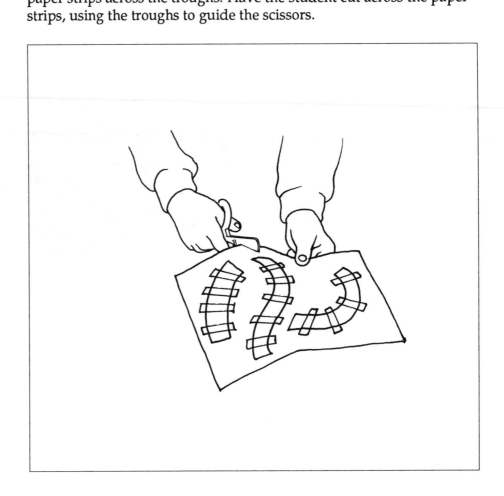

■ Classroom Scissor Activity

Purpose To teach the student to control the direction of the scissors (cutting curved lines)

Scissor Skill Level Stages 7, 8

Materials Paper
Paper punch
Scissors

Procedure Punch holes in a curve along the paper. Have the student cut along the curve, using the holes to guide the scissors.

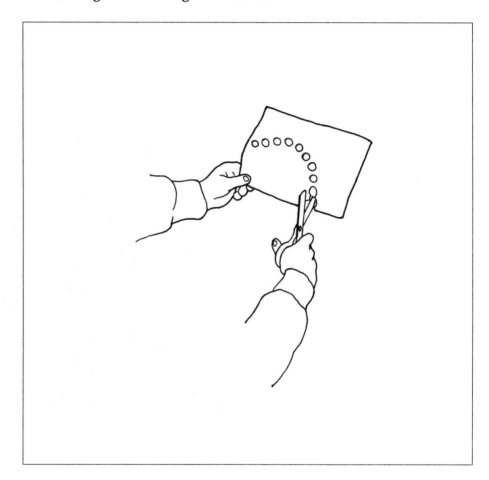

■ Classroom Scissor Activity

Purpose   To teach the student to control the direction of the scissors (cutting lines)

Scissor Skill Level   Stage 8

Materials   Paper
Pencil
Scissors

Procedure   Draw a circle on a sheet of paper. Draw lines to the circle, forming "sunbeams." Have the student cut off the sunbeams. By cutting small curved segments, the student successfully cuts out the entire circle.

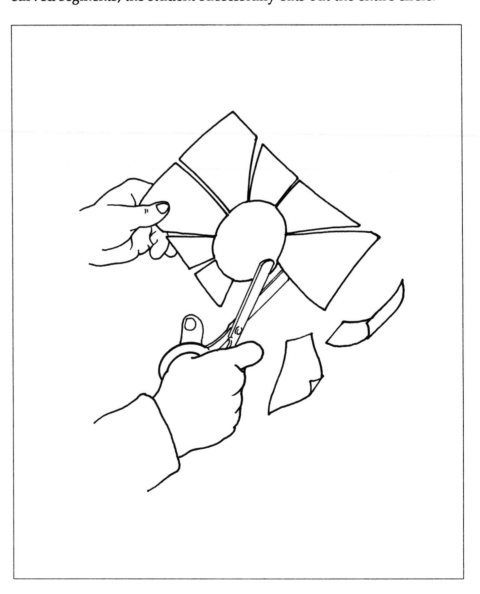

Classroom Scissor Activity

Purpose _____

_____

_____

_____

Scissor Skill Level _____

Materials _____

_____

_____

_____

Procedure _____

_____

_____

_____

_____

_____

_____

_____

_____

_____

_____

_____

_____

Classroom Scissor Activity

Purpose _____

_____

_____

_____

Scissor Skill Level _____

Materials _____

_____

_____

_____

_____

Procedure _____

_____

_____

_____

_____

_____

_____

_____

_____

_____

_____

_____

_____

_____

_____

_____

8 Individual Education Plans for Scissor Usage

We have examined prerequisites, developmental stages of scissor usage, and factors to consider in choosing appropriate cutting materials. Pre-scissor practice and classroom activities were suggested. Now you are ready to make this information work for you and your students.

Whether you devise an informal program or a formal written program to meet your federal, state, or local education standards, the following factors should be considered:

1 Long-Term Goal

What is a *realistic* long-term expectation for this student? Do you expect total independence in scissor skills, or do physical limitations indicate that semi-independence or adapted independence is more realistic?

2 Student's Sequential Scissor Skills and Abilities

At what stage or step of sequential scissor usage is the student currently performing successfully? Clearly indicate what the learner can and cannot do in scissor tasks.

3 Sequential Objective

Once the student's current level of sequential scissor skill has been determined, the next stage of sequential development can be assigned as the objective.

It is important to write the objective *specifically* and *measurably* in order to document progress and help the student succeed.

What is the specific behavior to be learned?

Is the objective learnable?

Is it broken down into small enough steps so the student can succeed?

Is the objective written in behavioral terms that can be measured?

What is the criterion for success?

How often does the task need to be performed successfully for the student to advance to the next step?

4 Methodology or Technique

How are you going to teach this behavior? Any methodology or task analysis should include these factors:

What the teacher will do or say to elicit the desired response (directions or cues to the student)

What the student is expected to do or say in response

The type of reinforcement that will be provided for a correct response (praise, or a tangible reinforcement)

What action the teacher will take if the student responds incorrectly to original directions (repeat directions? provide imitative model? provide physical assistance?)

How data will be collected

5 Environment

Where will the student sit when performing the task?

Are there any special positioning considerations to be made for the student's physical limitations? It is important for the student to be seated comfortably, so that attention can be focused on the task being learned rather than on balance or comfort.

6 Equipment

What specific equipment is needed to implement the objective?

What type of scissors is needed for the student to have maximum success?

Is a special weight or texture of paper needed to teach this skill?

7 Maintenance Acitvities

What type of activity will the student practice in order to maintain the new skill?

Individual Scissor Plan

Name _____

Classroom _____

Date _____

Long-Term Goal _____

_____

Sequential Scissor Skills _____

_____

Sequential Objective _____

_____

Methodology or Technique _____

_____

Environment _____

_____

_____

Equipment _____

_____

Maintenance Activities _____

_____

_____

_____

_____

_____

_____

_____

_____

Post-Test

1. **List ten prerequisites for cutting.**

    1._____

    2._____

    3._____

    4._____

    5._____

    6._____

    7._____

    8._____

    9._____

    10._____

2. **List the developmental stages of cutting.**

    1._____

    2._____

    3._____

    4._____

    5._____

    6._____

    7._____

    8._____

    9._____

    10._____

    11._____

3. **Name three types of paper that can be used in scissor practice, ranking them in the order of difficulty.**

    1._____

    2._____

    3._____

4. Describe three pre-scissor experience games.

1._____

2._____

3._____

5. List four factors to be considered when selecting scissors for an individual student.

1._____

2._____

3._____

4._____

6. Describe four (or more) types of scissors.

1._____

2._____

3._____

4._____

7. List three adaptations that can help a student who tears paper or bends it in the scissors.

1._____

2._____

3._____

8. Describe four (or more) adaptations that can be used to increase scissor control.

1._____

2._____

3._____

4._____

9. Name six (or more) classroom scissor activities that can enhance scissor coordination.

1._____

2._____

3._____

4._____

5._____

6._____